This book is dedicated to my husband Randy, mother May, and children Joel and Laura. Also, this book is for all the caretakers, everywhere!

I also wish to thank the friends who kept by me in the hard times and did not forget me. You know who you are.

Special thanks to my primary care health provider LNP Jeremy Waldo.

Very special thanks to the website NeuroTalk and the MTBI post-concussion syndrome forum.

"What's a Concussion?," and *"My Ghost Me"* were previously published in the *Rochester Post Bulletin*.

Copyright © 2014 by Jennifer Jesseph

Make Art From Your Splattered, Scattered Brain; My Journey Through Post-Concussion Syndrome

ISBN 978-1500646080
ISBN 1500646083

Cover art photography by Laura Torgeson

Self-published with CreateSpace

I0438199

Table of Contents

Introduction

On February 23rd, 2013, I was in a car accident and got a mild concussion. I was told at the ER I would be able to sleep it off, go to work Monday, and even enjoy some wine later that night. That was a lie.

My concussion healed some with brain rest, but the healing came undone, or it was never really done, because in March of 2013, I slipped into the world of post-concussion syndrome. This is a big word, but it means the doctors really don't know why your brain is still broken, and some of the doctors don't know how to help you either. There is still much that scientists are learning about the brain, and brain injury recovery is in the dawn of our understanding.

Today I find I have recovered a lot from light and sound sensitivity, daily dizziness, and extreme fatigue. I can count myself among the brain injury survivors. That said, I am still brain healing and I have invisible scars which manifest sometimes in struggling with oral language, loud sounds, and confusion if there is too much talking or activity. I do find humor with my struggles.

This book is a compilation of journals, poems, and dialogues about my healing from post-concussion syndrome. The book is intended for anyone suffering from this horrible affliction, caretakers, therapists, and medical workers who work with people who have brain injuries.

All our thoughts take energy, so I am working on feeding the good thoughts with positive energy.

This book is in chronological order, and the sections are short in case you have trouble reading or concentrating.

Can You Feel My Brokenness?

I have no cast
on my head,
or around my eyes
that pinch with pain
when I see those
hot pink, neon yellow, and orange colors,
but my brain is broken.

You can't put your hand
on the cracks,
but if you stay with me
and listen,
if you reach out your hand
I will take it in mine.

I will tell you how it felt
when my brain broke,
and I thought it was a joke,
a simple nothing, long headache
that would heal fast,
but it didn't.

Stay with me in these pages
and I will tell you one story.
My story, about a brain breaking
then healing,
and me, coming back to me.

Feel my brokenness
and if you do,
and have it too, I know
and I pray some day
others can really see it,
but for now they can only feel it
through our eyes.

Water Set to Simmer

The water filled pot
is on a cold stove.
I have to boil water.
Now, I have to remember
how to turn on a stove.

The pot waits
and I watch it
wishing it would simmer.

Early in my brain injury
I leaned into the mirror
many times
looking at my face.

*How can I look normal
and feel so odd?*

The pot of water
stays on the cold stove
for months.

I wait,
eat good food,
sleep, and sit
a lot. To anyone else,
I might look lazy
or crazy,
but I was neither.

This was brain rest.
I was the pot of water
on a cold stove.

All I could do was wonder if, or how
I would ever bubble back.

Saturday, Feb 23rd, 2013

Driving down Highway '52,
meeting mom for lunch,
then a walk at the mall. It's a clear day,
but yesterday we got 7 inches of snow
and had a late start at school.

As I drive, I talk to traffic
because that is what I do.
"Slow down sonny,"
to the big black pickup
roaring past me.

Cruise control is on
because that's how I drive when the highway
is clear and dry.
I hate speeding.

I notice a white car in front of me,
left lane, fast lane, slowing
and going left into the median.

"Someone is sick?
No exit there."

Whooshing crash,
I pull hard to the right.
MUST BE ICE! MUST BE ICE!
Oh ACCIDENT!!
Down I go
into the ditch,
those 7 soft inches of snow
cushion, and I am in shock.

White car, man in it,
up ahead in the ditch,

WHAT HAPPENED?

Two women, my angels,
stop and tell me
the white car sideswiped me,
and they wait till the police come
to file a report.

I refuse an ambulance.

Iamfine, I say fast,
ReallyIdon't wantanyambulance.
My head is feeling bubbly,
but I am fine. Chatty.

It's cold, so I take out
my boots from the trunk
and put my bright pink tennis shoes away.

I blanket one of the angel ladies
who is cold,
teeth chattering,
and we talk. I talk fast

because it's cold,
and I am in shock,
I think,

but I don't know yet
how sick I am.

Monday, Feb 25th, 2013

First day
back at work
after the accident.

Sometimes I st st sttuutter
when I ttrryyyyyy too ttttalk
and I never did
before.

Worked, teaching
all day
with a brain injury,

felt broken in my mind

like a CD that skips,
chips in a china plate,
something was amiss,
amok, and I felt it,

I didn't know how to say

"My brain is broken,"

and according to the ER doctor,
I'd be fine
like a glass of wine,

and I looked good,
but inside I was wood
or splinters
and smashed shingles.

My husband took me
to my regular doctor
because I had a pain in my chest,
pulled muscle.

A student nurse is writing notes
and I tell her I am laughing
all the time
even if something isn't funny,
          it's funny to me.

But if I laugh
the problem will go away,
I think. That's how it's always
worked before
and I am going to laugh away this brokenness.

Brain is fuzzy
and everything's funny,

Doctor: You have a concussion. You can't work. No Screens. No
TV. No Computer.

Me: No work? Whhhhhhhhaaaaaaaaaattttttt??? The ER doctor said I
could work!

Doctor: NO WORK FOR THE REST OF THIS WEEK. NO
SCREENS. WEAR SUNGLASSES IN THE HOUSE. YOU
HAVE TO REST YOUR BRAIN!

Me: But I have to work…………..

Doctor: N.O. WORK for the rest of this week. You'll come back to
see me Friday, and then maybe half days next week.

Me: (I am silent. Now I have more sub plans to make. I've already
been so sick this year. More sub plans. Oh God.)

Doctor: You'll have to get other people to get your sub plans ready.
You can't ride in the car. It's too visually stimulating.

Me: (My mind is wandering, thoughts are like shredded rags whipping in the wind.) (I am trying to figure out sub plans) (Doctor has no idea I have to write the plans. There is no one else at school doing what I do. He's clueless about that, and I have no idea either..........that I)

Doctor: NEED BRAIN REST. He tells my husband about a concussion he had once from football. He was knocked out, doesn't remember being brought back to the huddle, and to this day, things are rewired differently for him. Can't remember lines from movies, lyrics of songs.........

Me: (I am trying to figure out brain rest) OK I'll stay home and knit.

Doctor: N.O. YOU NEED BRAIN REST!

Me: I'll read a book.

Doctor: NO! NO! NO! YOU HAVE TO REST YOUR BRAIN.

Me: (silent, my rag thoughts try to gather and reform, but lay limp)

Doctor: And NO EXERCISE.

Me: Not even for my shoulder? (I am in physical therapy because of shoulder surgery)

Doctor: N.O.

Me: WWWHHHYYY??? (I want to cry) His stiff words pounding,
                              sounding stern.
                              Blue eyes flashing,
                              very firm.

Doctor: You probably feel deflated right now.

Me: (Deflated? Yes, and crumpled up like a dirty paper plate. Everything's shifting and tilting and changing so fast. No laugh, laugh, laugh is going to fix this.)

Doctor: OK, you can do your shoulder exercises, but don't push yourself. Don't work anything to exhaustion. You have to rest your brain.

Me: BUT what about the ER doctor? Why did he say I'd be all right by today? Why????????????????????????? (And why is the world a little spinny all the time?)

Doctor: I'll have to have a talk with Peter in the ER. (Doctor is finishing up. I can see hear him talking to my husband who is my accurate eyes and ears now.)

In the end, I believe my medical doctor
because my laughy, spinny world,
my giddy funny me,

is really quite broken,
and if fixing is brain rest,
then brain rest it is.

Why Do I Look So Good?

I leaned into the mirror
looking at my face.
It was fine.

My clothes –
clean, professional,
my rings, and things
rounding out my work ME.

I look good, so I will feel better later.
Probably in the afternoon
or by tomorrow,
surely. Yes?

Oh, that dreadful hope,
that silly lie I clung to,
but it had been firmly planted
by that ER doctor.
"You can work on Monday."

Here was Monday,
and why could I look so good
and feel so dizzy
and out of my body
like I was watching a movie?

I would later find
this is called disassociation
or brain fog.
It's common with post-concussion syndrome,
but scary.

My ghost me
was beginning to inhabit
while my ME needed
to heal.

But I had no idea
of any of that.
Work was work,
and if I looked fine
then I would be fine.

That was always the mantra,
the law,
the essential way it worked for me.

But little by little
I crumbled that day
till I was all in,
washed up,
exhausted, brain exhausted
and injured,
and my exterior
was never going to show
the broken interior.

But I didn't know!

Until, my good, regular doctor
became upset
and was quite firm.

"YOU CAN'T WORK WITH A CONCUSSION!
YOU NEED BRAIN REST."

But even then
I couldn't quite see why
I would look so fine,
so me,
and feel so ill.

It didn't all sink in,
how sick I was and only I
could feel it and see it.

I had yet to learn to listen to ME
and demand the truth.
That ER doctor's nonsense
was a full blown tree inside
from the one seed
he planted.
"You'll be fine.
You can have a glass of wine."

I clung to that lie
for awhile,
until it all faded
and no amount of makeup
or silver jewelry
or that bad medical advice

could cover up the truth.

Looking good
was just confusing the fact
that I was not on track
to recover.

I was quite sick
with symptoms
I would have to decipher
for myself.

I would have to learn
to ask the right questions
to the right people
and learn to give up
the life I knew

so I might heal.
It was an ordeal.

A long fight with myself
because I didn't understand

my health
state was not like a broken bone
so easy to see
to chart, to fix
compared to this.

Concussion Sleep

Concussion sleep is unlike anything I have ever encountered before. Even the fatigued sleep that comes with the third trimester of pregnancy is nothing like concussion sleep. I remember it could come on very suddenly and sometimes it felt like mild nausea, but it was not sickness. It was a horribly deep and unsatisfying sleep.

One day, early in my recovery, I was in a store with my husband, and very suddenly I felt a wave of exhaustion come over me. There was no fighting through it. I had to find a place to sit down immediately. That wave was likely followed with one of the horrible crash naps which are part of brain recovery, but did not feel restorative.

Likely, if you care for a brain injured person, you know they sleep a lot. Honestly, they have no choice in the matter, and if their sleep was like mine, it just did not feel great on waking. If you are a fellow sufferer, then you know exactly how tiring and frustrating concussion sleep feels. I recall it well, and hope never to feel it again, and I hope you'll be finding yourself in better brain days to come.

Concussion Sleep

Concussion sleep
grave bed deep
Felt like sickness.
Muddled me heap.

Came in a wave.
Must lie down.
Concussion sleep.
Afternoon drown.

Never a dream.
Waking, felt worse.
Concussion sleep.
Brain healing curse.

Why aren't I better?
When will this quit?
Family can't peace me.
I can just sit.

Brain makes me sleep.
This sleep is no good.
I wake feeling tired.
My mind, rotten wood.

Waking up mean,
and lashing around.
"Turn off those lights.
Quiet! No sound!

Choke back your happy.
Get out of my way.
No, you can't help me.
I hate me this way."

Crash napped me
didn't yet know
brain healing's tired.
Brain healing's slow.

Brain healing happens.
The nap was a sign,
I wasn't yet better.
I was far from fine.

Concussion sleep.
Ugly and deep.
Restorative? No.
Awoke feeling slow.

Woke up spent
and not feeling well.
Caught in a trap
of broken brain hell.

Crash Naps

Crash naps happen
with brain fatigue.

You know that weighted feeling
coming,
no avoiding it.

No drug,
no energy drink,
no exercise,
will stop this
steam roller sleep
barreling
toward you.

"Push through those naps,"
said the neurologist.
"It will help you
sleep at night."

She's never been
in the path of this monster sleep
that WILL OPEN it's warm
mouth, swallow you whole
into its belly

because your brain
is plain
worn out.
OUT of commission,
UNDER construction,
UNavailable,

and YOU are about to succumb
to its knock out punch,
its drag you down, down

deep
to ocean sleep.

No dreams
in a crash nap,
just a wicked deepness
that can last two hours
or twenty minutes.
On waking,
I often felt worse.
Not rested.
No zing of refreshed sleep.
No uplifting, sunny bright yellow balloon.
No jumpy, recovery, happiness.
No.

Just a heavy,
foggy, warm and muggy,
tropical slowness
pervading my mind.

I am in S L O W
M O T I O N
after the crash nap.

Fast words or cracking wit
just make me sad
or prickly with irritation.

Waking is like being in molasses,
thick and thickening.
My words are morass
and if I try to be fast
I just slow down

to sit on the couch,
or a chair,
or anywhere
away from noise.

Nothing to do
after a crash nap
but wait till dinner,
and then more time
to pass
till bedtime
and more sleep.

Journal: Friday, March 1st, 2013

I returned to work this week. I had a good, full day.
I felt play
and words were within me.

We went out to dinner,
daughter, husband, and me.
It was sweet
to eat out.

The concussion felt healed
and I was better.

The evening air was winter crisp
and cold
but a hint of spring
or something
warm lingered.

It was March
and the start of a new month.
Spring would come soon
and the moon
was waxing
toward good things.

We got Laura's track shoes
and some purple pens.
I was so glad
to feel better.
I could knit
a sweater
or do most anything.
I had mended.

But really,
it had not ended.

Got the flu.
Some sickness came back
and I was dizzing
and dizzy
and wobbly
in my mind.

I was gone from work three days
for illness.
And then,
worse things happened.
The lights were always too bright
and looking at pure white
was awful.

The diamond, glittering snow
I love and know
made me sick to see.

Oh, what is happening to me?

My regular doctor referred me to a neurologist
and I knew this was not good.
My splintered, wood mind
was back.

Doctor: You'll need a CT scan of your brain.
There's not much more I can do for you.

Me: Outwardly I nod and mumble agreements. (Inwardly I am
thinking, afraid and I want to cry.
But why? You can help.
You knew about brain rest. You helped me then.
Why not now?

Doctor: You need to see a neurologist.

Me: (Thinking and scared) This was a parting,
and I knew it. I could see the doctor shrinking away

because he's smart and knows
when he must bow out
and let a specialist decide.
He's smart, that doctor.
He doesn't let pride
rule. He knows when
he cannot take you further.
Even if I prefer him
over others, he knows
what he doesn't know.

And at that moment
I had no idea
how much I didn't know
or was about to learn.

For now it was sounds and light
and skull pain
all from a broken brain.
And I needed to sleep
at so many different times.
My sleep did not make me
feel better.

It was the slow, sad, slide
down
into the unknown,
uncharted,
uncertain dark waters
of

post
    concussion
        syndrome.

What is Post-Concussion Syndrome?

It's another big word.
At its essence it means this.
No one
knows
why your concussion healed
then unhealed
and you get the horrible
invisible symptoms
of headaches,
photophobia (light sensitivity),
hyperacusis (sound sensitivity),
big ugly fatigue (yuck),
vision problems,
finding it hard to be with people,

and the list goes on.

Your broken brain stew.
So what can you do?
There is no quick fix
that will mend broken you.

Reduce all your stress.
Give anger away.
Rest and be quiet
for many a day.

Some vitamins, supplements
help with that stress.
Do I take those?
Oh yes, yes, yes, yes.

Drop out of work.
Drop out of school.
Some friends will drop you.
Yeah, it's not cool.

Brain healing's slow.
Takes weeks maybe years.
No one can say
no matter your fears.

Your brain can heal.
It's slow. That's true.
Give it its time
and you will be new.

What will be new?
You will find out.
Maybe you're loud
and like to shout.

Maybe you're quiet
and can't stand a crowd.
You used to be bold
and lively aloud.

Maybe you're happy
and revel delight.
My awe is now deep.
My joy is kite height.

So strap on your patience
and buckle in calm.
These, my friends,
will be your new balm.

Dear brain broken people,
I write this for you.
Believe in brain healing.
Believe it. It's true.

Brain Rest

The first time I ever heard of brain rest was during teaching at school. Another teacher was commenting that a student had a doctor's note saying she was on brain rest and needed minimal stimulation in order to heal a concussion. That teacher and I scoffed at this idea. Little did I know that one day I would become quite familiar with brain rest. To this day, I wonder why that student was even at school trying to brain rest.

Brain rest was completely confusing to me. I remember sitting in the doctor's office and one by one every single thing I thought I could do to rest was quickly shot down with a blunt, "No! You can't do that!" It was utterly frustrating. For the first time I felt like I was being rapidly stripped of who I was as a person. I was not allowed to drive, ride in a car, read, knit, crochet, write, or think. Imagine being told you can't do any of your usual or beloved activities until further notice.

Even today, people new to concussion healing on the message boards or at NeuroTalk sometimes underestimate the importance of leading that very dull life of brain rest. But it is essential to brain healing, and if you do it right, you will help yourself down the road in recovery, and you might just avoid the nightmare of post-concussion syndrome.

My goal in writing about brain rest was twofold. First, I wanted to illustrate my brain rest experience. Second, I wanted to offer ideas of what you can do during brain rest. This, I hope, will help my fellow sufferers endure this time a bit better, and it might offer the gentle caretakers ideas of what a brain injured person can do during this time.

Brain Rest
for J. Waldo

Once you're brain sick
you'll ask, "What can I take
to make
this awfulness go away?"
The good doctor will say,
"Nothing, son.
Go home and rest your brain."

No screens, no texting,
no reading, just resting.
No movies, no TV.
You've got to believe me!
Your poor broken brain
needs just rest.

Just sleeping
and chilling.
You have to be
willing
to let yourself
really get rest.

No driving.
No working.
No quick movements, jerking.

And please son,
believe me,
you really must
heed me,
your brain needs
it quiet.
No anger,
no riot.

No alcohol drinking,
no parties,
no thinking.
No worries,
no hurries.

No hard exercise.
No fun for your eyes,
just rest, rest, rest, rest,
rest, rest, rest
YES!
Brain rest.

What You Can Do During Brain Rest
for J. Waldo

Pet a dog or cat.
Feed some fish
and watch them swish
in water.
Wait.
Just wait a lot.

Put your fingers
in dirt.
Plant seeds
in little cups.
Notice, each day
what comes up.

If it's summer
go outside and feel
grass under your toes
or between your fingers.
Lay down
on a lawn and listen
to your heart beat.

Run water in a tub.
Watch water
fall and feel it.
Pour in something soothing
and soak.

Take a short walk
if you can stand the sun.
Wear sunglasses
and don't run,
just walk.
Look at the trees
and listen to them sing.

Even in winter
They have songs to bring.

Listen to stories
on CD, or radio.
But if it tires you
or you can't follow
the story,
then just let it go.

Try classical music
if it's not too loud.
If the high pitches
or cymbal crashes
make you wince,
then quit.

Watch birds
from your window
if the light's not too bright.
See squirrels
swirling around trees
with their amazing tails.

Lay down
on your living room floor
and count your breath.
Think only of breath.
Not sadness,
pain, or death.
Breath is life.
Life is dear.
Breathe in your hands
and feet.
Find the right beat.
Just breathe.

Untangle some yarn
or roll it in balls.
Let it slip around your
fingers
and think of the invisible
threads of your brain
repairing.
It happens when you're sleeping
or staring away.

Fold socks, shirts, pants,
and any laundry.
Feel each texture
as you fold.
Let the cloth
tell you the stories
it might hold.

Sort a deck of cards
and shuffle them too.
Play solitaire.
If that makes you tired
or wired then stop.
Go lie down
and rest.
From your bedroom window
watch trees
bend in the breeze
and learn to bend too.

This is brain rest
and some things
you can do.

Please Don't Forget Me!

Healing from a brain injury is lonely. There was so much of the world I couldn't bear being around. Shopping under fluorescent lights was so tiring that I had to rest all morning just to make it for an hour or less in a big store.

But the loneliness was also palpable for me. I couldn't go to work and see people I enjoyed.

For a month I wrote substitute plans, but all that thinking work wore me out, and made me more lonesome for the work I did as a teacher.

When I finally realized I would not be able to finish the school year, I felt relief, sadness, and a huge loss. I've worked at some kind of paying job since I was sixteen. And now, very suddenly, I was unsure if I would ever go back to work.

> Lonely, lonely,
> bored, bored, bored.
> Wish someone would call
> and tell
> me something
> from work
> or, "How are You?"
> which is the hardest most layered
> question to answer.
> And who wants the REAL answer?
> It's long, and complicated
> like many balls of yarn twinned
> together.
> At the time I was most ill
> I had no words,
> no metaphors,
> no rhyme,
> to explain my very bad time.

Also my answer
was invisible
because any well wisher
who has never
had a brain injury or been invisibly hurt,
has almost no point of reference,
though some will try to understand.

At least I found people online
who knew and understood
this invisible affliction.
I found hope there too.

My work place
mostly forgot me.
I asked for a get well card
and I got one,
but it wasn't a genuine
get well. It was just a card
that I asked for.

If you have an invisible injury,
it's hard understand
that you are sick.
It's a trick
because your brain is you,
and if your brain is sick
how can you understand?

But my workplace
mostly forgot me.
They didn't mean to.
I've done that too—
just moved on,
when a coworker is gone.
I had my own
very busy, supercharged
world to watch.

But I was very sick,
and few called or cared or knew.

It's how it goes
when no one knows
or can see
the injury.

We have to use words
which I can use now.
At the time
it hurt too much to write,
think, or create.

Though I understand why
I was forgotten,
it still felt rotten.
I treasure the real people
around me now.
They shine like jewels.

Brain Rest Was Boring

And I hated it. I listened to classical
music on the radio
until the violins were humming too hard
in frenetic high pitches.
I lay in bed listening to audio books.
I went in and out of sleep
and no dreams.
I listened to the TV.
Sat with my back
to the screen
hoping I'd feel better
tomorrow
and tomorrow
    and tomorrow,
but so many times
I woke up in the morning

brain tired.

And I knew I was in for a long day
of staying away from the eye cringing white snow,
just being indoors,
in my curtained rooms,
before the sun soaked
everything in light
too bright for me.

My Energy, March 2013

When I woke up in the morning
I almost felt better and I could mistake this for
that slippery, elusive word. Recovery.

But I knew better.
This was no recovery. It was just the first energy
of the day,
and no one could say
for sure how long it would last,
but this is what it was like.

I felt good, but still tired.
It was like a cotton blanket
covered me. So, by 9 A.M.
I knew I could knit, or read a little,
but by 10 or 11:30,
a flannel blanket
was over my head.
I could watch TV
and eat a salad lunch.
By 1:30, a wool blanket
was covering me, pulling me down
into the crash nap
and there was no way
to work through that impending sleep.

And this was what a normal day was like
for a few months.

It made me scared.
I wasn't sure I could ever work again.
No one can promise you healing
from post-concussion syndrome.

I had to wait, hope,
and learn patience.

Symptoms of Post-Concussion Syndrome

The brain is often compared to the hard drive of a computer. I will use this analogy as I can't find a better one. If your hard drive is damaged, then any number of problems can arise from your computer. The same thing is true of your brain. Since your brain controls every aspect of your body and life, if it gets hurt, then so much can be affected.

The following list is by no means exhaustive. Here are some of the symptoms of post-concussion syndrome. Headaches, light and sound sensitivity, difficulty being in crowds, difficulty following a conversation, extreme fatigue, confusion, dizziness, issues with smell, and eyesight.

When I look back at my symptoms and compare mine to others, I know how lucky I was. I had a few headaches early on, but not daily headaches. I did have daily dizziness for a while which was cured with vestibular therapy. I also had hyperacusis and tinnitus which can still flare up. I also had a lot of difficulty being around people, following conversations, and short term memory lapses. To this date, I can still become very tired after very exciting events and I need to rest. Also, my tinnitus starts singing when I am very tired. If I am around very loud music with a lot of stimulation going on, I can feel physically sick or exhausted the next day.

I am glad to report, however, that most of my symptoms are gone and things that remain such as confusing words or mixing words up just makes me laugh now. It's my deep wish that any fellow sufferer will feel relief from their symptoms as well.

Insomnia

Lack of sleep
       so deep.
I can't let myself
find dreams again.

I wake up
and don't let myself look
at the clock
for fear
the time
is not enough.

Brain injuries
can cause insomnia.

Cruel.

You'd think
brain injured people
who need sleep
would just naturally
always sleep
and find peace.
Or, that they'd be
in deep, dark medicine sleep
as for for bone surgery.
Well, that's not
how it was for me.

One awful side effect
or full effect
of brain injuries
can be lack of sleep.

Insomnia.

Here is a snapshot of **Me** and **My Broken Brain**
trying to sleep after waking at 2 AM,
knowing I work must work
in the morning.

Me: Relax, tune out. Think of nothing.
Hear the pulsing sound of the washer.
Thumb, Thumb, Thumb.

My broken brain: Thumbs, --thumbs up for yes,
Thumbs down for no. Right students? Hush. Hush.

Hush a bye baby
on the tree top.
When the wind blows.

OH NO! That baby's going to fall and get a brain injury. How was
that song ever figured to be a lullaby? I guess anything is a lullaby if
you sing it softly.

Nursery – I think I have nursery duty at church. I will have to see.

Now
I have two plant nurseries inside.

Me: Relax. Think of nothing. Hear the furnace's white noise music.
Hear the washer going: thumb, thumb, thumb.
Quiet mind. Think of breath. Count your breath.

My Broken Brain: Breath
What rhymes with breath? Death, meth, theft. Theft is internal
rhyme. Does that count?
Remember to count. Count.
One, two, three, four, five, six
                              pick up sticks.

Me: Relax. Think of nothing. Hear the furnace's white noise music.
Hear the washer going: thumb, thumb, thumb.
Quiet mind. Think of breath. Count your breath.

Impulsivity

It starts with an imp
and bursts
right out of my mouth.
Wham! Wham!
Like a hammer
pounding.
Or, it pops and explodes
like gunshots
with my unedited,
> unvarnished,
> unkind,
> > unasked for
> > > thoughts.

My words blurt
bullet fast,
can hurt people
in their path
and leave us all
sorry.

My impulsive me
bought a blueberry bush
the first day I could drive
twenty five miles
and attend a retirement party
all. by. myself.

Later, I read the tag
and it said the bush
could grow to be six feet.
Oops!
We planted it anyhow
and ate those semisweet
berries last summer.

Photophobia
dim the lights, no spotlight, please

Sensitive to light.

The fake lights
in a big box store
made me run
for real, softer,
natural light.

I couldn't look
at stark white
like the blinding
brilliance of snow.
No. I would wince
and look away.

I needed sunglasses
inside stores
and out of doors
to keep the light at bay.
I needed
darkened rooms
like caves, or tombs
to rest my brain
from that light.

In time
colors came back
as their own,
real hues.

What's there to do?
Rest your brain
and wait.

There's no pushing past
photophobia

which by its root words
means fear of light.

For me,
that was never right.
I need the light
as it returns
from winter's long darkness.
I never feared light.

I LOVE colors.
Bring me that fuchsia pink
with some glittering violet.
Mix those colors.

I can see most colors again,
except bright neon orange
and neon yellow in fake, florescent
lights, are too bright for me.

Will that leave
and go away?
Or is photophobia
here to stay
in some way?
Who can say?

Only me.
Only time
has taken away
most of that
photophobia,

but some light sensitivity
still lingers around
and I wonder again,

what was mild
about that concussion?

My Scattered Brain

My scattered brain
so splattered brain
the thoughts are chugging
like a train.

I'll try again
and try again

to organize this
scattered brain.

My MTBI is like this.

It's as if three large file cabinets
opened each drawer
and barfed out all my manila folders,
the papers,
pencils, paper clips
everything went out.

Paper is everywhere now.
It's on the floor,
ceiling,
windows.

Some of the files are gone.
Lost forever.

Other files I can gather up,
replace, and resort,
but it's going to take months
or years.

So, when I forget your name,
or appointments,
or the day, or the reason I called you

or when I forget my words,

and when I buy blueberry bushes
that might become trees,

or I am distracted by bees
and hives and honey,
or I get to wondering
about cloud pictures,
and staring at shadows
and sun spots,
or I act wild
like an impulsive child,
and my thoughts just swirl,

this is my
new life.

My strife,
my struggle,

my MTBI.

My scattered brain,
my splattered brain.

My thoughts are chugging
like a train.

HYPERACUSIS
SHHHHHHHHHHHHHHHHHH, whisper this poem.

Big word for sounds
even music you loved,
is just NOISE and it can hurt you
to hear it.

Sounds I could not stand
when my post-concussion syndrome
was in its full bloom…

silverware clinking,
or unloading the dishwasher
if I did it at all
took time so I didn't knock
the dishes together.
The noise
of someone opening a bag of chips,
oooooooooooh such a cringing ouchy sound.

The loud WHACK THWACK
of a big knife hitting the cutting board
sent me far from the kitchen.

One evening,
while we had dinner in the darkened kitchen
to accommodate my light sensitivity
my mother knocked over
a jar of jam.
WHAM.

I had to leave
into my dark, cave room
alone. Too many sounds
already that day
made me tired.

Emotionality

I've always been an emotional person
and the brain injury
knocked out some and sometimes all
of my ability
to read a situation
and match my feeling to it.

Emotions.
The stuff of writers,
poets and painters.
That's me.

Emotions came back
at times and would rack
though me
and leave me surprised.

Like a child, (they are small people)
how emotions affect them.

The three year old who has a tantrum in the store
feels grief
flails on the floor.

I know that feeling too.
I try to keep it in check

but since my brain is still healing
some of my emotions
make me act a wreck.

Like the two year old who is overwhelmed
by lights, noise, music,
and they tell us
by falling asleep
or screamful tears.
So too, my injured brain does that to me

sometimes, and I can't always control it,
but I try.

It's not cute
when an adult
is overwhelmed
then falls asleep
in a chair.
It makes the other adults
wince
and aware
and wonder

WHAT'S WRONG WITH HER?
WHAT DID SHE SAY?

It's just my emotions
got the better of me
today.

But hey!

I can see it and I know.
I can feel it and I see.

I am getting better
which means
more healing
is happening.

I need to be very quiet
and chill
and silent
and still

and the rest of my Mes
are coming, coming back to Me.

Confusion

"Wait, what? What did you say?
Wait, were you talking to me?
What? What?"

How am I so lost
in all these people talking?

I am a lone, still fish at this party
among all the fast swimmers.

The fish above me
wiggle, wiggle slide
so easy, easy glide.

Their banter
is fast
but I am hushful
by my rock.

I watch them slipper,
slipper around
and past me.

"Wait, what? What did you say?
Could you repeat that?"

I can't keep up.

Other fish dart
from bottom to top
top to bottom
and whirl around
one another
in dizzying circles
of words
and jokes.

Me, I stay near
my rock
and try to think
about just one voice.
One conversation.
But I am in an ocean
of words,
and I just

can't keep up.

"What? Wait, what? I didn't hear that. Sorry."

When all the laughter
and cacophony of words
bubbles over
I know it's time to leave.

I swim back home
to my dark, cave room
with no voices
and no fast words
zipping around me.

Just calm, blank
silence.
At last.

Lost in Walmart

Why am I in the soup aisle?

Oh I am trying to remember
and all the cans
their shiny red, yellow, orange
labels

dis
     tract   me.   *"Whatever became of
Libbys Libbys Libbys on the label label label?
Oh, gluten free soup. What's that?"*

Oh no, here comes a lady with a big CART FULL of food
and children spilling everywhere….. How does she do it?
She's the young woman in a shoe,
                              and I am
wondering……….

Why am I in the soup aisle?

OH NO………………….. This store is going to swallow me.
The ceiling and floor are really a mouth and I need to get out.

all the BrIgHt florescent lights are cutting into me,
eating my energy,
making me sick,
and that dizzying, ugly, horrible monster feeling is rising up
and I know I must

get out of the soup aisle.

I walk quickly past
all the nauseous lime green fluorescent shirts,
and bright pink jittery pants.
These colors are killing me.
Get outside!

I have to feel
the air.

I find a tree in the parking lot. A lone tree,
and some grass. I can wait here,

breathe, dream, and maybe recall,

Why was I in the soup aisle?

Spring Cast Party, May 2013

"Hey, how
are you?

"Did you know
they are separated?"

I'm in the middle
of a swirl
of conversations,
people eating,
glasses clinking,

"Jojo, over
here!"

and I can't keep up
with multiple voices

"She's playing
guitar with
a new band."

and all the talking.
It's all too confusing,
brain diffusing,
not so amusing!

"Everyone knew
she would
get fired."

"Can I get you
a drink,
Jack?"

I can hear someone
telling a joke.
I laugh on cue, but why?
I didn't get it. Did I?

"He's the best
nurse."

I have to leave
get out into the real air,

"I got all
my cues
tonight."

away from garbled,
mind muddling voices.

"That last
scene....."

Donny, the Brittney Spaniel,
greets me on the back step.
It's almost midnight.
I scratch her ears
and watch stars
winking in the spring night.

The voices inside that made me dizzy,
float away.
I can feel Earth's heartbeat.

The dog, me,
and the night air.
This is where
I might find
a patch of peace.

Getting Help on the Internet

Recovering from post-concussion syndrome is by far the most isolating and lonely experience I've ever had. The internet was truly a life line to other people who had the same issues I had, and also to stories and people who were healed. The internet was a pipeline of hope and without it, I probably would have figured I was crazy or that I needed therapy. As it turned out, belonging to the groups that I did on Facebook and at NeuroTalk gave me the therapy I needed, and these groups still give me opportunities to help others as I was once helped.

If you are a young person with post-concussion syndrome, I hope you can find others like you to talk with, cope with, and get some ideas of how to live your life. There is a group for teens with post- concussion syndrome on Facebook and there are likely other groups available too on other social media networks. I encourage you to look into these groups.

Finding people like me helped my recovery immeasurably. It also lightened the burden for my family who could only understand to a point what I was going through.

No matter where you are in your journey with post-concussion syndrome, I really hope you are getting the care and therapy you need. I can't underscore it enough how important it was for me to connect with like injured people.

The following poems came from discussions with others on line about our symptoms, and our questions in general.

Bubbling

"A watched pot never boils"

Even so, I watched
and waited for water to boil.
I waited for bubbles
to dance to the surface,
break water's skin
and live free in the air.

So too, I waited
for myself
to emerge.
I never knew
if I'd bubble back
as me
or quite differently.

When the brain is hurt
there is no guarantee.
It's a time to wait,
watch and see.

Hopefully, quietly,
patiently,
I prayed I'd bubble
back as me.

Invisibly Injured Internet Friends

Invisibly ill people will
listen to others
on the internet

even if they are invisible.

Why? Because
the flesh, human doctors
or medical workers
don't know all the answers
about our broken brains.

You too
might turn to invisible answers
such as prayer,
meditation,

and anything that helps
when medications fail,

and you see your bright orange life
going pale,

and you are desperate to live
for your sons, your daughters,
your lovers, your life.

Invisibly injured people
will seek answers
anywhere.

Even the air,
from a ghost,
or a prayer.

We hope to find
someone kind.
Someone who can
help us.

We are all
desperate for answers.

Scary? Yes.
But when answers are
in short supply

invisible ones,
even if incorrect,
will do.

Owls and Dialogues

It's the middle of the night
and I can hear owls hooing outside my window.
Somewhere in the pasture
they whoo hoo hoo hoo
back and forth and back and forth.

It's comforting.
I can't sleep anyhow
so their hoos are better
than the traffic
or music.

Like owls hooing,
we with invisible inflictions,
so too, we hoo
to each other.

We are saying, "*I am here!*
From my tree
I can see
headaches, and endless days
of fatigue. What do you
see brother? Whoo hoo hoo hoo hoo?"

At this perch
I can see the sunrise
in my longer walks.
My dizziness has left
and something healing
is taking root. What do you
see sister? Whoo hoo hoo hoo?

I am down low
and afraid. When will it get better?
I used to run and pump iron.
Who am I now?
Whoo hooo hooo hoooo.

On and on
back and forth in our
mighty hoos
we tend to one another
and try to guide
those who want to give up,
or have doctors
who don't listen.
We minister to them

and our echoes of hoos,
our words out there,
might help others
who want to remain
in the shadows,
hooless, nameless,
but they can read
our dialogues
on the message boards.

Those owls,
those silent ones,
we hope you listen
and *whoo hoo hoo hoo*
if you can

and we will *whoo hoo hoo hoo*
back
to let you know
what we see
from our tree.

Broken Glass

Everyone I know
with post-concussion syndrome
is broken.

Some of us are smashed bottles,
slivers and bits.

Some are bottles
with jagged ridges
and a base in tact.

Some – holes
punched through
panes of glass.

Or, like a broken windshield
with a tangled web
of glass lines.

Some of us
are in so many chunks
and pieces
all over the place.

We, the broken glass people,
feel our way around
trying to find our bits.

Everyone is asking,
How can we fix
this brokenness?

We ask each other.
We cry out!

"Please! Help me find
relief from this headache

light sensitivity
all this noise!
The crowds and the talking
are making me sick!!"

We wait and look
for the medicine,
the fix,
the cure,
the way to wholeness.
We are all
trying to mend
our broken glass,

and no one
knows
when, how, or if

we will fix.

So, we just wait
in this shattered
crushed
minced
way.

We wait,
and with our words
we help one another.

Some days, we feel better,

and sometimes

we just stare and sleep
in shatteredness.

Return To Play

What's that mean for the football
who is two years out with sound and light
sensitivity and begins each day
with a headache?

Return to play guidelines.
First concussion.
May return to play after a WEEK
if the symptoms are gone.
Second concussion.
May return to play in TWO weeks
if all symptoms are gone.
Third concussion.
Terminate season.

Terminate return to play
is what I say.

Oh those young men, all ID,
all frontal in the head.
How they want to get back
to the team,
to the great, big adrenaline rush,
to the life.

It's cruel
saying, "It's just a concussion.
You can get back, Jack.
Just rest and it will all shake off."

They can cling to that lie.
But this is the truth.
Every time you break your brain
you make it weaker.
Every brain injury makes it more
likely you'll get another.
Sorry brother. Time to be blunt.

You want to avoid
post-concussion syndrome
which, if you get it, means this.
You won't return to play
that game again. Ever.

So, you're sidelined,
but who needs to be sidelined
are the owners who pressure players
to heal faster. "Come on! Get out there! Perform.
We've got your clean uniform."

Sideline those guidelines
giving false hopes
to the brain injured.
Sideline these words forever.
"It's just a concussion."

Just ask Pam, Olympic skier,
who passes out daily
during exercise.
Two years this way,
and she's still asking,
"When can I return to play?"

Ask Kevin,
professional snowboarder
until his massive TBI
hospitalized him for a month.
Upon coming out of his coma,
he asks, "When can I snowboard again? When?"
He keeps asking, and every time
his mom's face crumples
like wadded paper.
He can't see himself,
how broken, how injured,
how he has no balance.
His injury has left him a shadow,

a shell, and it's his shell
he will have to reconcile.

Return to play?
Return to pray
is what I say.

Every day I pray for people with brain injuries.
Especially the young people
who have so much life left.

There's no more return to play.
Not that way.
What more to say?
That dream, that life
must float away –
maybe meld into something new.
Only your new you can say.
Until then, just return to pray,
for each day
and just one day
at a time.

How Are You? Late May, 2013

Wow, that question
used to blew me away
back in days
when I couldn't figure out
what to say.

Should I tell them the truth?
That honestly,
I feel brain broken?
But back then
I didn't even have those words
in mind, or in my mouth yet.

Should I lie and say "Fine,"
like people do all the time
even if they are not.
There is no time
to really tell anyone
how you really are,
unless you do have time
with them.

Here's how I did answer
when I tried to be back at work
early in brain recovery
and I wasn't fine,
but needed a quick answer
because in America
we like fast answers,
and fast medicine,
and fast fixes.

Fast Answers for HOW ARE YOU DOING?

I'm doing my best.
I'm doing.
I'm well enough. (This was a lie)

I'm not great.
I'm not all there.

In late May, 3 months post accident,
my doctor asked me,

HOW ARE YOU?

He was taking a nettle out of my thumb
and my foggy brain was there.
It was misty and a strong sun
was peeking in through my thoughts
while I watched the doctor with large magnifying glasses
that could see the tiny thorn
in my thumb.

When that doctor asked
in his gentle way,

How are you?

it made me worried.
A tear of sweat dripped
down my back.
What are you asking? I wondered.

I partly panicked.
Was his question a riddle?
I didn't have the words to ask the doctor
to reframe his question.

So I said,

You know I'm not working, right?

Much later I realized of course he knows I'm not working.
He sees all the reports from the neurologist,
and knows.

But he doesn't know what was a blow
this concussion, and post-concussion syndrome
was for my husband, me,
my whole family.

Here's the answer I wanted to give
the doctor that day.
 I feel crushed,
scared, yet proud I drove myself to an appointment today.

I feel tired every afternoon. So, I'll leave soon
and have a long crash nap.
Doctor, do you know what that's like?
It's not fun.
But your just taking a nettle from my thumb
and your gentle question
"How are you?"
leaves me quite dumb.

Me: What am I to say? I ask my wandering mind.

Mind: The doctor asked, "How are you?"

Me: *Actually, pretty awful, worried, and feeling better too. I am walking more.*
I walked in a store and I felt better.
I mean, the florescent lights in the store didn't bother me too much.
And such and such and such.

Mind: I don't think he wants to know all that.

Me: What does he want to know?

Mind: How are you?

Me: Oh.

I could never be sure.

WHAT DID THAT QUESTION MEAN?

The appointment ended well enough,
but that question,

How are you?

is so tough
because it is so large,
and I always want to answer it
as honestly,
correctly,
and as concisely
as I could.

The answers to the big HOW ARE YOU?
have changed
as I have become better
and quieter,
or my louder me
is back again.

The question HOW ARE YOU
is really an invitation to everything and nothing.
It's a meaningless string
of words we bead together
to find out WHATEVER.

My brain injured me
sometimes stumbles
through visual and auditory cues.
Nuances of language
can be completely lost on me.

Such a LARGE question
as HOW ARE YOU?
can make me feel dizzy
and distracted, like looking at clouds
or that color of fire green in summer grass.

I'd rather it be like this.
Ask me the real question you want to know.

How is your brain feeling?

What's it like inside your head?

Have you been having better days since your accident?

Some might find this blunt,
but I like that direct question.
It narrows it down
to the brown bones
of what you want to know.

Don't make me guess.
Sometimes, I really can't.

And if you want to know how I am,
then please
make time for a nice long answer.
Make time
for tea and cloth napkins
and a long, sweet talk
like on a summer walk
because it's only fair.

If you ask ME that question
you may get a long,
whimsical
befuddling
funny
and honest
 answer,

and I will want that
from YOU too.

My Ghost Me

She –
in that picture-
she loves the sun.
See her squinting
and waving?
She could run,
and read books for hours.
Who IS she?
Not me.
Certainly,
not me now.

She is my Ghost me.
She once knit
a dress from pink wool
she bought in France.
She spoke French
and loved to rhyme.
Once upon a time,
she was me.
Oh, my Ghost me,
does some part of you
still live here now?

My New me
is not yet she.
Who is she,
this New me?
She's slower
and slowly
repairing her brain.
Will she be the same?

She can't yet say.
It's enough to live
and breathe in the day.
My new me knows this.

"I am enough today. I am enough."

My new me is quiet, and waits.
Sometimes she feels Ghost me stirring.
When the day is right
they just might
sing a duet.

Being Defined by a Brain Injury, December, 2013

"I won't let this define me!"

Some people say this
when met with their
adversity.

As for my brain
injury,
it's too late.
This injury already has
defined me.

My attention span
is as small as a flea
or a fly,
and I wish I
could fly
like I did in dreams.
Do you see what I mean?

Distractions
come easily.

And so does awe.
I am amazed
by shadows,
or sunlight
in windows,
or the blue hues
of snow
in January.

I can't keep hold
of hot anger
for long.
Because some song,
or memory of verse

will distract me
from the energy eating,
consuming feeling
of mad.
Anger's just bad
anyhow,
so I can give it away
and go on with my day
and forget whatever
blew up
or blew over
or blew by.
Good bye maddening anger.
Good bye.

A brain injury
also defines the family
when I have less tolerance
for noise,
or I get brain tired
and my concussion naps
come back.

"Turn down
the volume on the TV!
It's not for you,
but for me.
That sound
is too much
too loud
too big
and it hurts my head."

Poor family
has to live in the defines
and confines
of a brain injured person.

They don't always like it either.

It's a drag
being around me
if I get tired
and need a rest.
Oh family, you do
your best
and put up with me
and I you.

It's what we have to do
for now
for a while
or a long time.

But I have faith
and the healing feelings
are coming more.
No one knows
what is in store
because
those horrible symptoms
can come back.
I've lived that.
So, life is day to day,
and hope and pray
and pray.

The brain injury
has made me different
and somehow new.

I won't wish it on anyone.
Neither would you.

June 2013, Conversations

I used to be so good
and talking to everything.
I could make talk
out of nothing
and everything,
and now

talking is thinking,
and thinking is broken.

So, conversations
and people
can tire me out.

Some talk is overwhelming
and I never know why
or when it might happen,
but I can feel my brain

sssllloooowwwiinnnngggg
dddddooowwwnnn

and becoming distracted
by words,
or what someone's wearing,
or light from a window,
making a shadow
on the floor.

I try to pull myself
back once more
into the threads
of the story,

but I can't always
manage to understand
where the conversation
is going.

I can fake a laugh, smile
and sort of be in the loop

for awhile,
until I simply have to stop,
and leave because
all the talk
is making me tired
and sometimes sick.
What's the trick?
I wonder.

I look good, have been feeling
better, and yet,

conversations,
people talking,
and people
can make me very tired.

Recovery from MTBI

Recovery. That is one tricky word. Usually, it connotes being symptom free and healed. It is a word we can use to ultimately describe being free from the illness, or brokenness that plagued us and we can now live our lives as we once did.

Recovery from a brain injury, from my experience, is not like recovery from the flu or healing broken bones. In brain healing, I say that I live in a state of recovery, which for me means that some of my symptoms can recur and this is something I have to learn to live with. For example, if I become overly excited by cheering hard at a track meet then I can get light headed and feel weak. If I have too much exciting stimulation like being at a wedding and talking to many, many people, then again I might get a light headed feeling. When I work too long on my computer, or if I knit or read for an extended time, I can feel really tired and need a break from these activities. I assure you this is different than how I lived before, but any time I feel discouraged by it, I only need to recall the awful days of needing that deep, unhappy sleep for eighteen hours a day, and I no longer feel discontent.

But I don't want to scare anyone who is still struggling with their symptoms more than a year post accident. There is still so much unknown about brain healing and we do know that the brain heals very slowly, so please, stay the course and hang in there.

Ironically, I think I am now the healthiest I have ever been in my life as I live in recovery from a brain injury. I love to walk outside and I can walk for hours on a sunny day. I enjoy planting flowers from seed and weeding my flower gardens. I am careful about what I eat. I do eat a lot of fruits and vegetables, and I can't drink much alcohol anymore, but that is a very small thing to give up in order to maximize health.

I am living a full life where I can work, and I really enjoy writing and all kinds of creative activities again. If I have a bad brain day, then I know it was just that. It was one bad day, and it won't last.

I feel quite hopeful as I look forward to the future where I think I will have the best and the rest of my life back.

If you are still seeking answers for your symptoms then I hope you keep searching. There are many remedies available now that I didn't need, but others have benefitted from these, and science is still working to uncover the mysteries of the brain. There is reason to be hopeful.

Recovery

Recovery,
that slippery word
like trying to hold a Sunfish
you caught with your bare hands,
but its flippy, fishy bones fight you
and it you can't hold it.
The fish goes free.

Slippery,
like black ice
that sends cars spinning
on the highway
and into the ditch.

One good day
in brain recovery is just
one good day, and nothing more.

To recover,
don't hover
over the past when you could push
yourself to the MAX.
Learn to link the good days
together gently, slowly,
without weeping and worry,
or the flutter and flurry of trying to go back
to exactly
as you were because you THOUGHT it was finally OVER.

Hush yourself.
Be gentle and try to walk,
but don't exhaust.
        Just exhale.

No head pounding hard workouts. No.
Stretch out easily
and in quiet places.

If you OVERdo it and try to go back
to that fast track of who you were, multi-tasking,
                                    multilayered
lists, texts, hyper-quick, super energy charged life

you might only
set yourself BACK
further

and you will need your curtained rooms
to dim the bright lights again
and more rest.

Recovery
takes unknown amounts of time
with brain injuries.
If you are lucky
you can learn to listen
to your body
and respect its limits.

Or, the body
will enforce
its limits with headaches,
extreme fatigue,
brain fog,
and more.

Recovery,
that slippery word
we can't use in brain healing.
When your brain's better,
you may live in recovery.
Keep your days free of stress
and watch out.
Some symptoms may come back.
The tinging ear ringing returns
when I am so tired.

Brain fog creeps in around fatigue.
And confusion,
or fear of fast traffic alarms me
sometimes.

But mostly
I am better and better
and I live
in a recovery.
My recovery.

You have to create your own recovery
and listen to how it will
frame your days.

What's Mild about a Brain Injury?

Really? MTBI.
Mild Traumatic Brain Injury.
How is it ever mild?

Mild is a balmy 72 degree temperature
in July with light breezes
stirring whipped cream clouds in a blueberry sky.

Mild is a sweet, zingy salsa sauce
that won't burn your tongue.

Mild, is easy
like falling in a leaf pile,

or watering my coneflowers
or watching my impatiens bloom.

What is mild
about a brain injury?

Nothing.
Zilch.
Nada.

Just ask Quinn
whose headache starts
every morning as a hum,
becomes a drum, then roars
in her head like a firey sun.

Ask Aaron who used to work
in a high tech computer job,
triple fast multitasking, e-mails,
calls, textes with his thumbs,
fast zip, fast tick tick tick,
doing thinking going
all the time.

Now, he's relearning division
and multiplication.
Conversations
make him tired.
He hasn't worked
in two years.

Ask Ellie
who looks drunk
when she walks.

The only thing
mild about a brain injury
is how we are treated
from this invisible dilemma.

We get mild, blank stares
if we try to tell you
that harsh fluorescent lights
can make us sick.
We might look drunk and giddy,
but really
we just can't always
control ourselves,
because our brains
are broken.

Mild is a word
that must make doctors
feel better
when they have no idea
what to prescribe
for our dizziness,
the horrific headaches,
the severe sensitivity to sound,
the insomnia.

Mild,
really describes the medical minds
that think we are just making up all our symptoms
because we need attention.
Oh, those doctors are mild.

Brain injuries mild?
No.
Never.
Nada.
Zilch.

Quartet for MTBI

Mild

Breezy,
quite easy.
But this
word is crazy.
It's an absurd
word
to describe any
brain injury.
Mild's just
not quite right,
but I am polite
and will let it go
even though
I know
there is nothing
mild in describing
a broken brain.

Traumatic

Scary! Blue, red, white
lights flashing.
Sirens whining, crying.

Traumatic
is the last gasp
before the woman on the high wire
falls,
or when you pull hard to the right
to avoid another car crashing
into you.

Traumatic
is rapid heartbeats

and you wake up sweating
and not forgetting.
Why does it seem
so real?
When your so scared
you can't speak,
it's traumatic.
Traumatic
is afraid, always
and lives in the coldest
place in you.

Brain

Computer,
Chief Executive Officer.
Creative Director.
Beautiful Being.
Dream Holder.
My Inner Card Catalogue.
Every Picture Album.
Container of All My Days.
My Sun and Moon.
The Circuit Box.
The Mother Board.
Harbor of my Soul.
Me.

Injury

Ouch
hurt
broken bone
broken heart
broken brain

Wound
won't heal.

Bruises
black, blue
yellow.

Blood splattered.
Dislocation.
Decapitation.
Severed hand,s
       legs,
        fingers.

How We See Someone Is Injured

Wheelchair
catheter
heart monitor
bandage
cast
bruise
slings
crutches
wires
braces
limp
cane

Invisibly Injured

I use words
metaphors
and similes
to compare
my pain
to what you can see.

Sometimes,
 I speak anew

or I make up words
or I misfire
when I talk.

It's hard to explain
for the brain

of the invisibly injured
can be mental pain

you can't see
but we know

we are not right,
or all there.

Sometimes
my injury
makes me laugh.

It used to make
me cry,
and sigh,
and wish.
and wonder,

and wait,
to get better.

Become a Recovery Artist

Trapeze artists
dive toward one another,
hand to hand,
swoop to swoop,
swing to swing,
somersault,
never falling,
always moving.
They catch
and catch
in grace.

This is my life
in brain
recovery.

When sounds
are too loud
I volley forth,
and swing away
from cringing noise.
I can disappear
in midair.

When I can't
follow the threads
of conversation,
it's not my imagination.
I somersault swirl away.

When bright flashing lights,
and traffic
whirring past
make me dizzy,

then I close my eyes,
reach out

and grasp
the hands that catch
and pull me
to dark velvet quiet.

This is me
now. I'm a recovery
artist who can
disappear
in a whirl.

I am she
who will reach
and catch herself
before
it becomes too much.

I reach to reach,
catch to catch,
and know when
to bow out,
and
vanish.

Brain Food

Avocado, avocado,
purple grapes.

Green leafy salads.
Strawberry shapes.

Brown rice, brown rice,
lentils, eggs.

Farm fresh meat
like chicken legs.

Sweet potato, sweet potato,
spinach too.

Watermelon, watermelon's,
good for you.

Pineapple, pineapple,
salmon, fish.

Oranges, apples.
All you wish.

Blueberry, blueberry,
nuts, flaxseed.

Eat well! Heal well!
You'll succeed.

Yogurt, yogurt,
not too sweet.

These are brain foods
you can eat.

Brain Healing, Like Watching a Baby Grow Up

The baby's first year
from learning to feed,
finding their feet, and hands,
creeping, walking
to talking,

is a marvelous evolution
of change.

Healing from a brain injury
was also an evolution.

In the early months
I was like a baby.
I demanded what I needed.
My demands were not always harsh
but they commands
and a source of survival.

"Turn down the loud music.
Those high pitched violins
are hurting my ears.
Please slow down the car.
I can't take this fast driving.
Please go slowly over bumps.
My head is whirling
and I am sick."

In a few more months,
I could do more,
like a two or three year old
who has figured out a puzzle.

Then, my teenage me
appeared with her blunt words,
her impatience,
and impulsivity.

She embarrassed herself at times
and later wondered,

"What did I just say?"

Finally,
when the laughing,
really happy, giddy me
came to live
back in the brain
and the body,

I knew. I was brain healing.

Giddy me
can laugh at her mistakes
with joy.

Happy me is the one
I choose over all the others.

Come Happy Me!
Dance in the living room again.
Listen music
and just throw up your arms.
Embrace the healing feeling.

Happy me
is she who loves children.
It is she who loves
her husband,
best boyfriend ever.

When happy me
is here, the world
swirls with night stars.
It tips over sweetly
with a great laugh
and a sigh.

Happy me,
I didn't know
when or how
you might appear,

Stay for now,
forever, and just be

like a content
baby sleeping.
Be the cool of the evening
after a long, humid
day.

Happy me,
please stay.
It was for you I waited.
For you, I prayed.

Praise for my Caretakers!

Dear husband of gentle hands,
driving me to doctor appointments,
taking notes and keeping track of me.
Maker of colorful salads!
Gentle reminder, "Don't get greedy," you said once
when during one good day early in brain recovery
I wanted to proclaim "RECOVERED from post-concussion
syndrome," but I was not. It was just one good day.

Thank you and bless you for all your patience.

Dear daughter,
fetcher of water,
you tucked me in many times.
Dear remover my reading glasses
when I fell asleep too tired to move.
Dear sweet talker, telling me of your day
and helping me play word games.
You helped my loneliness go away.

Thank you and bless you for your patience.

Dear mother,
best designated driver,
bringing me to work on the weekends
when I tried so hard to return to teaching.
"Just one more week
of sub plans." But I was wrong.
You always waited so kindly.
Gentle listener, and helper,
even when I snapped
in anger at the concussion.

Thank you and bless you for your patience.

To All Caretakers Everywhere!

I am so grateful
for your care.
You made me aware
of how much I needed you.
You were the glue
that helped me heal.
That was for real.

I thank you
and bless you.
What more can I do?
If you are sick
or feeling frail,
I'll help you.
I will never fail
to be your caretaker too.
This is love, and true.
It's what we must do.

We are born to help
each other.
This is the lesson,
the beautiful gift.
One another
we uplift
and help be whole.
That is the goal.

Thank you and bless you,
caretakers, all.
Your gift is remembered.
It was not small.

You made life bearable,
even when I was cranky
and terrible,
and weary, and full of despair.

It's your care
that pulled me through.
Yes, that's true.
Your care pulled me through.
So thank you and bless you.

Post Concussion Style

I'm going out
for just awhile.
So, now it's time
for post concussion style.

First, sport my best,
soft ear plugs to reduce noise.
Or, have them in my pocket
just in case
noises begin to clammer.

Next, those fine
sunglasses.
Oh, something classic,
so I don't look tragic.

I am hopeful
for a short walk
around the block,
or to the park and back.
Just a short walk
to move my blood
and move me forward
another inch, or square.

Now, a nice hat
to cut down on the glare.
People may stare
and wonder why,
but you and I know.

It's our style.
Now, for awhile.

I need the air.
I need to see

anything besides my cave room,
it's dark, and gloom.

I have my phone
in case I feel lost
or need to talk
while I walk.

Last, I have water.
Plenty of water to keep
hydration going.

So, here I go.
It won't take too long.

I have my earplugs,
my dark glasses, and hat.
What do you think
of all that?

I am walking away
from my dark room.
Just for awhile
in my best, most sexy
post concussion style.

Math Facts

Subtraction

When the ER doctor
asked what is 45 minus 15
I snapped, "It's a number!"
At that moment
and for several months
after the accident, subtraction
was hard, even impossible for me.

Dear daughter,
that brain sickness subtracted
me from your Junior year
and made prom dress shopping
unthinkable.
The day we went to the mall
and I suffered those sickening
fluorescent lights while you
slid so easily from store to store
finding dress shoes,
I subtracted myself
from your shopping to sit,
rest and wait.

I was minus you
and daddy when I could not
attend plays.

Dear son,
my broken brain withdrew
 me from your competition ballroom
dance. I won't lie.
I did cry, staying home.
Not even a poem
made me happy,

but it was too tiring
to feel very sad.

The brain injury
subtracted me from events
I once enjoyed,
rendered me a fraction
of who I was,

so I holed up
in my dark rooms,
away from noises
and overwhelming conversations.

Addition

Addition started dully
with adding one brain tired
day to the next,
and waiting to add another
in hopes that a glimmer of better
was in its dawn.

Slowly,
addition began to grow
when I could walk a mile,
then a mile and a half.
This took a few months.

Adding the days
where I could do more,
and drive a little further
without becoming exhausted
was hopeful.

Then, in June,
addition burst into multiplication
of miles I could walk and drive.

When I could finally subtract
the afternoon crash nap
from my life
I knew I was multiplying
three digit numbers.

The good days
kept adding up
slowly and sweetly.
When humor and word play
returned, it all added to me
till I became almost
a whole number again.

What's a Concussion?

Concussion

Almost rhymes
with cushion
which sounds fluffy
and floofy
like your head was hit
with feathers
or wind.

But that's a lie.

Concussion
per the dictionary:

Violent shock,
jarring, jamming,
organ injury
such as the brain,
which may result
in a long loss of function.

Concussion

Troubling word,
not a verb,
but a painting word
describing your brain
in pain
when it's been shaken,
stirred, and hit so hard

that some fine wires
break in there,
but no one can see
because no camera

no MRI is powerful
enough to show
the blow,
the hit
the bad break.

The word concussion
means nothing
to me anymore.

Let's give that word away.

It's really
a brain break.
it's a hurt,
        wound
        sore, tear, lesion--
an invisible injury
that hurts.
It was cracks in my mind
that drained me of life.

Dreaming Again!

Dreams swam back
on some rainy nights
in October, 2013,
and my world held not just color,
and all manner of lights (fluorescent, sun, light bulbs,)

and dreams again!

Crazy dreams
making little sense
and problem solving dreams
where I process solutions.

Dreams.

For seven months
I had no dreams
I could recall.

So many dreamless,
dull nights,
like gray, cloud filled days,
or plain oatmeal
every. single. night.

But, as colors came back,
and noise became music again
so too, dreams returned
in their own time,
not my time.

They flickered
to life,
  awakening,
   harkening,
   singing.

Dreams swam back
from their deep canals.

Dreams!
The sweet fruit
of slumber.

Those fragments
of folly,
or amusement,
or puzzlement.

Another sign
of a mind healing,
             restoring,
             repairing.

Another rejoicable moment!
A gift to behold.

No one's too old
for the peace
of dreaming.

Oh dreams!
You awaken
my thankful me.

I feel
my creative,
zig zag, lemon yellow,
electric life --

my poetry me
is surely home
and filling
my mind again.

Living In Recovery

Some things are definitely different now that my brain has pretty much rewired. Basically, I feel like every day is a new chance to do things and to make dreams come true. I use writing, knitting and crochet as ways of self expression. From where I sit now, life is just more fun and funnier. I know I laugh more now than I did before my brain injury.

If you are recovering from your own injury, I hope you are bubbling back as a happy person. We can't control what we can keep or lose from the injury, but with time, it's my belief we can control how we will feel and react. It's our job to embrace the new people we become and learn to carry on as best as we can.

Words Keep Bubbling Back

Yes, she wrote that feeling
funny and spill giggly. That was when words bubbled
back so fast they spill mixed
with other words and blended
to the pinks and purples
of coming summer skies
that May lets free
when humidity
gives off a huge **HUFFF**
and a **PUFF** and blows winter
away, away, away.

It was this night, and gorgeously,
when her daughter sang
her last choir concert
of high school.
So many voices she knew
and knows and the words
bubbled again and again
and words bubbled in tears
and joys and no fears.

Just one large sigh of
mint and forest green.
Such peace.

A year ago all those sounds
were just noise.
Killing, hurtful noise
in a brain injured woman
who loved music but the music
made her sick, and mad.

The ugly holes in her brain
must be healing
because such bubbling
and spilling, and free mixing

of giggling pink and sweet smiling
orange are here again.

She can hear again
and she celebrates this night
and every night with feeling
smile giggly
smile giggly
glittering fuchsia kissing sweet orange
blessed.

Ebullition

The state of bubbling up.
Good sweet joy
bubbling over,
drenching into
the parches of dry, bald
drinkless soil.

Ebullition.
blaze, burst burst burst
of amaze, amazement, amazing,
joy, joy, joyness, of fire cracking,
firework brilliant, awe felt joy.

Ebullition.
A gushing wind storm
of words, and word finding,
word play, playing words,
and connecting back
to people
to love
to life.

Ebullition.
A rapid frenzy, frenzy
of feelings, gushing, rushing yessing
and all good good glorious
yes yes yesness to being alive.
An explosion
of liveliness, of life,
when you know the rapid pulse
of the earth and every human
is in you
and this world is the gift
and I can feel it again
and I live.

Ebullition.

Fishing on Muddy Lake

My broken brain
was a long drag
down to the bottom
of Muddy Lake.
I sank deeper
and deeper each sick day.
Down the swirling,
chocolate waters,
with no compass,
no bearing on the sun,
and no way home.
I sank with nothing
but prayer to guide.

I dropped down
to the muddy bottom
and let silt bury me
in its tar depth.
This was death,
but I was alive.
I saw nothing,
dreamt never,
and prayed
despite my despair.

Slowly,
I started to come up.
At first,
I felt the silt lift,
then I could swim a little.
Weeds swished past me
and fish fins fanned
my arms and legs.

Sometimes
I fell back, down
toward the mucky bottom,

but I didn't get trapped
there again.

Every day
I tried to swim a little farther,
                         up, up, up.
The water became clearer
and clearer
until one day

I broke the surface
and breathed air again.
I knew then,
I was on the way home
to my ME.

It took months,
but I finally got out
of Muddy Lake.
Now, I live outside
that water.

I look out at Muddy Lake
where I lived/died/lived,
where I prayed so hard
and God heard me.

He lifted me up,
slowly, gently,
                 deliberately,
and breathed life into my being
so I could live once more.

I stand on the shore
and skip rocks
to the center of Muddy Lake,
the place that took me down,
where I left my ache.

But I am here now!
Cartwheeling free! Full of sun vigor
and joyful smiles!
My hands are full of pink impatiens,
fresh red raspberries, and apples
for anyone.

Here I am!
See me sing and spin!
I live and rejoice!

I AM ALIVE!!

I live and feel peace.

I live and these lines
are my strings of hope
for you,

if you have
some sickness too,
or you are hurt

or lost

or feel despair—

I am casting out for you.
I care!

Here come more lines.
Reach out!
Catch my words
and I will reel you in.

Neuroplasticity Cheer

Neuroplasticity
That is the word for me!

Neuroplasticity
That is the word for me!

Neurons connecting
with one another.

Nerves can communicate.
"Hi I'm your brother."

Wires, wires, wires, wires
communication.

Neurons, neurons, neurons, neurons
send information.

Wires, wires, wires, wires
eyes to the brainy brain.

Neurons, neurons, neurons, neurons
react in a chainy chain.

Does the brain stop
once its done growing?

Is it all done
with all its knowing?

No! and Yea! No! and Yea!

Neuroplasticity!
What's it mean for injury?

Neuroplasticity!
What's it mean for injury?

Brain can reorganize!
Make new connections.

Brain can reorganize!
Neuron selections.

Brain can reorganize!
Maximize the function.

Brain can reorganize
over damaged junction.

Undamaged axons
grow new nerve endings.

Undamaged axons
help in brain mendings.

Undamaged axons
link with a mystery.

Undamaged axons
help with brain injury!

Neuroplasticity
That is the word for me!

Neuroplasticity
That is the word for me!

Make Art From Your Splattered, Scattered Brain

Let it rain. Let it rain. Let it rain.

When you're sad, feeling strife,
wonder what's the point of life?

Watch the moon. Paint the sun.
You have only just begun.

Go outside. Feel the air.
Art's alive and everywhere.

Let it rain. Let it rain. Let it rain.

Oh, it's hard. It's not fun.
Is brain healing ever done?

Broken brain. Headache pain.
Life is down the muddy drain.

Wonder why, and you cry,
"Who am I? Who am I? Who am I?"

So make art from your splattered, scattered brain.
Let it rain. Let it rain. Let it rain.

Deep sadness makes you stew,
feel there's nothing left of you,

all the music that you knew
makes no sense, leaves you blue

and the friendships that you had
fade away, makes you sad.

Let it rain. Let it rain. Let it rain.

Art's in everything we do.
Take a walk. Tie your shoe.

Dance upstairs. Fry an egg,
Pet a dog. Stretch your leg.

Knit a scarf. Mold some clay.
Oh allow! Time to play!

Just make art from your splattered, scattered brain.
Let it rain. Let it rain. Let it rain.

Don't give breath to all your pain,
or the loss of so much brain.

Hurt and tired all the time,
and it's difficult to climb.

Take the worries and the stress.
Make some art from scatteredness.

Let it rain. Let it rain. Let it rain.

My mind is made for rhyme,
and I like to let it chime.

Metaphor and poetry
are what make sense to me.

I hope you like it too,
and I wrote this all for you.

Just make art from your splattered, scattered brain.
Let it rain. Let it rain. Let it rain.

Journal topics and activities for those with a brain injury.

Use these topics to explore your own feelings about your head injury.

1. Who is your ghost you? Does that person haunt you from time to time? Write a letter to that ghost and reintroduce yourself as who you are now. Ask that ghost questions and see if there is any reply.

2. Early in recovery it was very hard for me to write much of anything. Can you list some of the things you can do? Look over the list from week to week or month to month so you can see your progress.

3. Write a letter to your symptoms. Introduce yourself and tell your symptoms how you feel.

4. Write a letter to a healthcare professional who has helped you. If you feel up to it, send that letter. Some never hear what they did right.

5. Write to the caregivers who help you. Maybe in your brain injured world, you might have taken someone for granted. Let them know your gratitude.

6. One way to brain rest is to work with your hands. Try knitting or crochet if it doesn't make you feel tired. Use YouTube to find tutorials that can help you. You might give painting or working with colored chalk or pencils too.

About the Author

Jennifer Jesseph lives in Pine Island, Minnesota with her husband and two children when they are home from college. She lives in a rural area with plenty of green space for vegetable and flower gardens.

She is working on her writing for children and writing poetry chants for teaching. You can find out more about her writing at her website and her author page at Facebook.

http://www.jenniferjesseph.com/

https://www.facebook.com/jenniferjesseph

www.ingramcontent.com/pod-product-compliance
Lightning Source LLC
Chambersburg PA
CBHW020541290526
45786CB00002B/985